NURSE LIFE

My Planner

○ MONDAY

PRIORITIES

○ TUESDAY

○ WEDNESDAY

TO DO

○ THURSDAY

○ FRIDAY

○ SATURDAY / SUNDAY

NURSE LIFE

My Planner

○ MONDAY

_____

PRIORITIES

_____

○ TUESDAY

_____

_____

_____

_____

○ WEDNESDAY

_____

TO DO

○ THURSDAY

_____

○ FRIDAY

_____

○ SATURDAY / SUNDAY

_____

NURSE LIFE

My Planner

○ MONDAY

PRIORITIES

○ TUESDAY

○ WEDNESDAY

TO DO

○ THURSDAY

○ FRIDAY

○ SATURDAY / SUNDAY

NURSE LIFE

My Planner

○ MONDAY

PRIORITIES

_____

_____

○ TUESDAY

_____

_____

_____

○ WEDNESDAY

TO DO

_____

_____

○ THURSDAY

_____

_____

_____

○ FRIDAY

_____

_____

_____

_____

○ SATURDAY / SUNDAY

_____

_____

NURSE LIFE

My Planner

○ MONDAY

PRIORITIES

○ TUESDAY

○ WEDNESDAY

TO DO

○ THURSDAY

○ FRIDAY

○ SATURDAY / SUNDAY

NURSE LIFE

My Planner

○ MONDAY

○ TUESDAY

○ WEDNESDAY

○ THURSDAY

○ FRIDAY

○ SATURDAY / SUNDAY

PRIORITIES

TO DO

NURSE LIFE

My Planner

○ MONDAY

PRIORITIES

○ TUESDAY

○ WEDNESDAY

TO DO

○ THURSDAY

○ FRIDAY

○ SATURDAY / SUNDAY

NURSE LIFE

MY GRADES TRACKER

Week	Monday	Tuesday	Wednesday	Thursday	Friday
1					
2					
3					
4					
5					
6					
7					
8					
9					
10					
11					
12					
13					
14					
15					
16					
17					
18					

Notes

NURSE LIFE

MY GRADES TRACKER

Week	Monday	Tuesday	Wednesday	Thursday	Friday
1					
2					
3					
4					
5					
6					
7					
8					
9					
10					
11					
12					
13					
14					
15					
16					
17					
18					

Notes

Made in the USA
Monee, IL
10 December 2019